# Dr. Sebi

MW00881482

## Diseases

The Ultimate Step By Step Guide On
Natural Treatment For Herpes, HIV,
Aids, Stds, Cancer, Diabetes, Erectile
Dysfunction, Arthritis, Kidney, And
Liver Diseases

By Margaret K. Ritz

**Legal Disclaimer:**

The information provided in this book is for educational and informational purposes only. It is not intended to replace professional medical advice, diagnosis, or treatment. If you have any questions about a medical problem, always consult your physician or another trained health expert. Never reject or delay obtaining competent medical advice because of what you've read in this book.

The author and publisher make no representations or warranties on the accuracy, applicability, fitness, or completeness of the contents of this book. They make no claims (express or implied), merchantability, or suitability for any particular purpose. The author and publisher will not be held liable for any loss or other damages, including but not limited to special, incidental, or consequential damages.

Any product names, logos, brands, and other trademarks or images used or referred to in this book are the property of their respective trademark holders. These trademark holders have no affiliation with the author or publisher and do not sponsor or promote this book.

# Table of Content

# INTRODUCTION

Every year, millions of people are diagnosed with illnesses that modern medicine claims to manage but not cure. In the heart of this global health crisis, Dr. Sebi's teachings as a self-taught herbalist from Honduras stand out as a beacon of hope.

Dr. Sebi's groundbreaking approach to health, which focuses on an alkaline diet to detoxify the body and treat the underlying causes of disease, calls into question the standard medical model, which frequently fails to heal. His concept, which focuses on reducing the mucus accumulation that he believes is the root cause of a variety of diseases, provides a simple and natural road to recovery and well-being.

## Dr. Sebi's Method Vs. Traditional Modern Medicine

While modern healthcare systems excel at emergency care and some therapies, they usually address disease symptoms rather than the root causes. This symptomatic strategy, which relies on medications, might result in a cycle of dependency and negative effects.

In contrast, Dr. Sebi's technique encourages a plant-based, alkaline diet that naturally supports the body's healing processes without the use of pharmaceuticals. His holistic perspective views health as a balance of body, mind, and spirit, advocating for a lifestyle that promotes all three for long-term wellness.

## How To Use This Book

This book is intended to be your guide and partner on the journey to greater health. Each chapter focuses on a different part of Dr. Sebi's therapy approaches, such as recognizing chronic conditions and putting his nutritional and herbal prescriptions into practice. You can read the chapters in whatever order you like or skip right to the sections that address your specific health concerns.

This guide is intended to introduce you to Dr. Sebi's healing principles and demonstrate how to apply them in your daily life for better health.

The Science of Healing: Learn why the body responds so well to an alkaline diet and the science behind Dr. Sebi's approach.

**Adopting the Alkaline Diet:** Learn about the major components of the alkaline diet, including which foods to eat and which food to avoid, along with meal plans and recipes.

**Lifestyle Changes for Optimal Health:** Discover how to apply Dr. Sebi's teachings in your daily life to reap long-term health advantages.

**Herbs For Health:** Learn about the herbal supplements advised by Dr. Sebi, including their purposes and how they aid in detoxification and healing.

## Who Is This Book For?

This book is for everyone looking for a natural, long-term solution to disease and health issues. It is intended for people who are skeptical of conventional medicine and wish to try a more natural approach to healthcare. Whether you're coping with chronic health difficulties, looking to improve your well-being, or are interested in preventive treatment, you'll discover excellent advice and practical solutions to help you navigate your health journey based on Dr. Sebi's concepts.

This book does more than just present an alternative; it provides a fresh perspective on health and healing, prompting you to reconsider how you approach your well-being. With Dr. Sebi's knowledge at its heart, it urges you to embark on a journey to a better, more vibrant existence.

# AN OVERVIEW OF DR. SEBI'S LIFE AND WORK

Dr. Sebi, born in Honduras in 1933 as Alfredo Bowman, was a self-taught herbalist, healer, and natural medicine advocate. His adventure into the world of healing began when he was diagnosed with asthma, diabetes, and obesity. Dissatisfied with conventional treatments that just treated symptoms, Dr. Sebi set out to seek alternative ways that addressed the underlying causes of sickness.

Dr. Sebi established a unique healing philosophy based on alkaline diets, fasting, and herbal medicines over the course of many years of research and testing. He thought that the body has an inbuilt power to cure itself when given the proper nutrient and environment.

Dr. Sebi's work received international notice in the 1980s, when he claimed to have discovered a treatment for AIDS, cancer, and other chronic ailments. Despite skepticism and criticism from the medical establishment, he remained committed to his holistic approach to healing, emphasizing the necessity of detoxifying and replenishing the body with natural, plant-based meals.

Dr. Sebi's theory revolved around the concept of bioelectric cell food, which he defined as food that is "consistent with the genetic predisposition of our bodies." He felt that eating alkaline-rich foods and avoiding acidic items might help restore the body's pH balance and promote overall health.

Throughout his life, Dr. Sebi was committed to sharing his expertise and empowering others to take charge of their health. He traveled frequently, lecturing and providing consultations to people seeking alternative health methods. His legacy lives on via the many lives he touched and the ideas he advocated for, motivating millions to adopt a natural and holistic approach to wellness.

In this chapter, we explored Dr. Sebi's personal biography, delving into the experiences and insights that shaped his healing philosophy. We also look at the key concepts of his method and how they might help us on our own path to robust health and energy.

## Dr. Sebi's Holistic Approach to Healing

Dr. Sebi's holistic approach to healing includes a thorough grasp of health and wellness that goes beyond simply treating symptoms. At the heart of his ideology is the concept that the body has a natural potential to repair itself when given the right nutrients and environment.

Dr. Sebi's holistic approach revolves around the concept of alkalinity. He highlighted the need to have an alkaline environment in the body rather than an acidic one. According to Dr. Sebi, many chronic diseases flourish in an acidic environment; thus, by alkalizing the body through diet and lifestyle changes, people can help their bodies heal naturally.

Dr. Sebi's treatment philosophy emphasizes the use of natural, plant-based meals as medicine. He advocated for a diet high in alkaline foods like fruits, veggies, nuts, seeds, and grains, and low in acidic items like meat, dairy, processed foods, and refined sugar. Consuming nutrient-dense, alkaline meals allows people to nourish their bodies and encourage maximum health from within.

In addition to dietary adjustments, Dr. Sebi stressed the significance of detoxification and cleansing to eliminate toxins and impurities from the body. He felt that fasting, herbal medicines, and other cleansing techniques may help restore the body's balance and energy.

Dr. Sebi's comprehensive approach includes addressing the mind-body link. He acknowledged the interdependence of physical, mental, and emotional health, emphasizing the need to maintain a good mentality and lower stress to promote overall well-being.

Overall, Dr. Sebi's holistic approach to treatment is based on the notion that true health is reached via balance and harmony between the body, mind, and spirit. Individuals who follow a holistic lifestyle that promotes alkalinity, natural foods, detoxification, and mental well-being can empower themselves to take control of their health and experience bright vitality.

# UNDERSTANDING CHRONIC DISEASES

## Understanding Chronic Diseases and Their Effects on Health

Chronic diseases are a broad category of ailments that affect many systems and organs in the body. Understanding the various types of chronic diseases, their underlying causes, and the consequences for health and well-being is critical for successful prevention and management.

**Types of Chronic Diseases:**

**Cardiovascular Diseases:** This area encompasses heart disease, stroke, and hypertension. Cardiovascular disorders are frequently associated with risk factors such as high level of cholesterol, high blood pressure, smoking, obesity, and inactivity.

**Diabetes:** Diabetes is a metabolic condition marked by elevated blood sugar levels. Type 2 diabetes, the most common type, is frequently linked to obesity, a poor diet, a sedentary lifestyle, and genetics.

**Cancer:** Cancer is a group of diseases/illnesses distinguished by the uncontrolled proliferation and spread of abnormal cells. Tobacco use, a poor diet, physical inactivity, toxin exposure, and a genetic predisposition all increase the risk of developing cancer.

**Respiratory Diseases:** Chronic respiratory illnesses, such as asthma, COPD, and bronchitis, impact the lungs and airways. Smoking, air pollution, allergies, and respiratory infections are all common causes.

**Autoimmune Diseases:** Many autoimmune diseases, such as lupus, rheumatoid arthritis, and multiple sclerosis, develop when the immune system misidentifies and destroys healthy cells and tissues. The specific causes of autoimmune illnesses are unknown, but genetic, environmental, and hormonal variables may all have a role.

**Underlying Causes of Chronic Diseases:**
Chronic diseases frequently have multiple causes, including a genetic predisposition, environmental variables, lifestyle choices, and socioeconomic determinants of health. Poor food, a lack of physical activity, tobacco use, excessive alcohol use, and exposure to environmental pollutants all contribute to the development of chronic diseases.

**Impact on Health and Wellbeing:**

Chronic diseases can have a great/significant impact on a person's physical, mental, & social health. Complications may include disability, reduced mobility, chronic pain, mental health concerns, and a lower quality of life. Chronic diseases also impose a considerable strain on healthcare systems, economies, and society as a whole, resulting in growing healthcare expenses, lower productivity, and higher mortality.

In conclusion, chronic diseases pose a significant public health challenge worldwide. Understanding the various types of chronic diseases, their underlying causes, and the effects on health and well-being allows us to better address the root causes and implement effective preventive, early detection, and management techniques.

## Common Chronic Diseases and Their Root Causes

Chronic diseases are common health disorders that continue over time and have a substantial impact on people's well-being. Understanding the most common chronic diseases and their underlying causes is critical to effective prevention and therapy.

### 1. Cardiovascular disease (CVD):

Cardiovascular disorders/diseases, including heart disease & stroke, are the leading causes of death worldwide.

**Root Causes:** CVD risk factors include high blood pressure, cholesterol, smoking, obesity, diabetes, and physical inactivity. These variables contribute to the development of atherosclerosis, which is the compilation of plaque in the arteries and can result in heart attacks and strokes.

## 2. Diabetes:

Diabetes is a metabolic condition/disease characterized by elevated blood sugar levels.

Root Causes: Type 2 diabetes, the most common type, is frequently associated with obesity, a poor diet, a sedentary lifestyle, and a hereditary susceptibility. Insulin resistance is a condition that make cells become less receptive to insulin, is a major factor in the development of type 2 diabetes.

## 3. Cancer:

Cancer is a class of diseases defined by abnormal cell proliferation.

**Root Causes:** Cancer formation is complex, with genetic abnormalities, environmental variables, and lifestyle decisions all playing a role. Tobacco smoke, UV light, and some chemicals are carcinogens that cause DNA damage and promote uncontrolled cell division.

## 4. Respiratory disease:

Chronic respiratory illnesses/diseases, such as asthma, chronic obstructive pulmonary disease (COPD), and bronchitis, have an impact on the lungs and airways.

**Root Causes:** Smoking, air pollution, allergens, respiratory infections, and occupational exposures all contribute to the spread of respiratory disorders. These variables can cause inflammation, constriction of the airways, and decreased lung function.

## 5. Autoimmune Diseases:

Autoimmune illnesses develop when the immune system erroneously assaults healthy cells and tissues.

Root Causes: The specific origins of autoimmune illnesses are unknown, however they may include a genetic predisposition, environmental triggers (such as infections or toxin exposure), and hormonal variables. Immune system dysregulation is important to the pathophysiology of autoimmune diseases.

Understanding the underlying causes of common chronic diseases enables people to make more educated health decisions and take preventive steps. Addressing modifiable risk factors through healthy lifestyle choices and early intervention can lessen the burden of chronic diseases while improving overall well-being.

# PRINCIPLES OF DR. SEBI'S HEALING METHODS

## Overview of Dr. Sebi's Principles for Achieving Optimal Health

Dr. Sebi's therapeutic methods are based on a holistic approach to health & wellness, emphasizing the body's natural ability to heal itself when you give it the proper conditions. Dr. Sebi's philosophy is based on five important ideas, which serve as the cornerstone for his approach to obtaining optimal health.

**1. Alkaline Diet:** Dr. Sebi recommended for an alkaline-rich diet made mostly of natural, plant-based foods. He felt that alkaline meals aid to keep the body's pH balanced and promote health and vigor. These foods include fruits, vegetables, nuts, seeds, grains, and herbal teas, while acidic foods like meat, dairy, processed foods, and refined sugars should be avoided.

**2. Fasting and Detoxification:** Dr. Sebi emphasizes the need of fasting and detoxification in his therapeutic methods. He felt that fasting allowed the body to rest, mend, and eliminate poisons accumulated from nutrition and the environment. Fasting can improve general health and well-being by resting the digestive system and facilitating the body's natural detoxifying processes.

**3. Herbal Remedies:** Dr. Sebi recommended herbal treatments derived from natural plants and herbs to aid in recovery. He felt that these botanical remedies had significant healing capabilities that could address specific health conditions while also restoring body balance. Herbal medicines are essential to Dr. Sebi's holistic therapeutic approach, from blood cleansing to organ function support.

**4. Electric Foods:** Dr. Sebi identified some foods as "electric" or "bioelectric cell foods" that align with the body's inherent biochemistry. These meals are often alkaline in nature and high in nutrients, vitamins, and minerals required for good health. By introducing electrified foods into their diets, people can fuel their bodies at the cellular level and enhance overall wellness.

In summary, Dr. Sebi's ideas for maximum health include eating an alkaline-rich diet, fasting and detoxifying procedures, using herbal medicines, and emphasizing electric foods. Individuals who embrace his beliefs and make lifestyle adjustments consistent with his holistic approach can assist their body's intrinsic healing capacities and experience increased vitality and well-being.

## Explanation of Alkaline Diets, Fasting, and Detoxification

Dr. Sebi's treatment approaches are based on the ideas of alkaline diets, fasting, and detoxification, all of which attempt to create an internal environment that promotes optimal health and healing.

### Alkaline Diets:

Alkaline diets aim to balance the body's pH level by consuming alkalizing foods. Dr. Sebi recommended a plant-based diet high in alkaline-forming foods such as fruits, veggies, nuts, seeds, and grains.

These meals are thought to nourish the body at the cellular level, giving important nutrients while also promoting detoxification and lowering inflammation. Individuals can maintain an alkaline balance in their bodies by avoiding acidic foods such as meat, dairy, processed meals, and refined carbohydrates, which Dr. Sebi believes is essential for overall health and wellness.

## Fasting:

Dr. Sebi believes that fasting is an effective method for healing and cleansing. By fasting for a set length of time, the body can redirect energy that would otherwise be needed for digestion into repair and regeneration activities. Fasting permits the body to remove toxins collected from diet and environmental exposure, enabling cellular repair and rejuvenation. Dr. Sebi advocated intermittent fasting as a way to rest the digestive system and boost the body's natural cleansing systems. Whether through intermittent fasting, juice fasting, or extended water fasting, fasting can help reset the body and boost overall health and energy.

## Detoxification:

Detoxification is the process of eliminating toxins and impurities from the body to improve organ performance and cellular health. Dr. Sebi's detoxification strategy entails supporting the body's natural detoxification pathways through dietary adjustments, herbal medicines, and fasting. Individuals who consume alkaline-rich meals and herbal teas can improve liver, kidney, and colon function, boosting the body's ability to eliminate waste and pollutants. Fasting also assists the body to eliminate accumulated toxins, whereas herbal therapies can help cleanse certain organs and systems. Regular detoxification techniques can help to support the body's natural healing processes while also promoting long-term health and well-being.

To summarize, Dr. Sebi's ideas of alkaline foods, fasting, and detoxification work together to create an internal environment that promotes healing and vitality. Individuals can support their body's natural ability to heal and prosper by adopting these practices and making lifestyle adjustments that are consistent with their holistic approach.

# THE ROLE OF NUTRITION IN HEALING

## Importance of Nutrition in Preventing and Treating Chronic Diseases

Nutrition is a crucial factor in the prevention & treatment of chronic diseases, as well as a potent tool for improving health and wellness. Dr. Sebi underlined the necessity of providing the body with natural, plant-based diets that promote maximum performance and vitality.

**Preventing Chronic Diseases:**

A well-balanced and nutrient-rich diet can prevent chronic diseases. Individuals can supplement their bodies with important vitamins, minerals, antioxidants, and phytonutrients by eating a range of whole foods such as nuts, fruits, veggies, seeds, and whole grains. These nutrients assist in improving the immune system, promote cellular health, and guard against oxidative stress and inflammation, lowering the chance of acquiring chronic diseases, including diabetes, heart disease, and cancer.

**Treating Chronic Diseases:**

Nutrition is vital for treating and managing chronic disorders. Dr. Sebi pushed for an alkaline-rich diet that eliminates acidic meals while including alkaline-forming foods to aid in the body's healing process. Consuming foods that nourish and alkalize the body can help to reduce/lower inflammation, increase nutrient absorption, and promote overall health and vigor. Furthermore, several foods and plants have been demonstrated to have therapeutic characteristics that can help relieve symptoms and improve outcomes for those living with chronic conditions. Garlic, for example, has been shown to improve heart health and lower blood pressure, whilst turmeric has anti-inflammatory & antioxidant properties that may aid people suffering from illnesses like arthritis or cancer.

In conclusion, the importance of diet in preventing and treating chronic diseases cannot be emphasized. Individuals can promote their body's natural healing processes and lower the risk of chronic illness onset by eating a plant-based diet high in nutrient-dense foods and including healing herbs and spices. Individuals can empower themselves to take total control of their health and experience increased vitality and well-being by implementing nutritional therapies that adhere to Dr. Sebi's beliefs.

## How to Follow a Dr. Sebi-Approved Diet for Optimal Health

Following a Dr. Sebi-approved diet is an essential component of his holistic approach to healing and achieving peak health. Individuals can nourish their bodies and promote their natural healing processes by eating alkaline-rich, plant-based diets and avoiding acidic foods.

## 1. Emphasize Alkaline Foods:

Dr. Sebi's diet emphasizes alkaline-forming foods to maintain body pH balance and promote health and vigor. These include fruits like bananas, cherries, and melons, as well as veggies like leafy greens, broccoli, and bell peppers. Alkaline grains such as quinoa and wild rice, as well as nuts, seeds, and herbal teas, are also recommended. Individuals can improve their overall health by focusing their meals on alkaline foods.

## 2. Avoid Acidic Foods:

Acidic meals are thought to cause inflammation, sickness, and imbalances in the body. Dr. Sebi suggested avoiding acidic meals including meat, dairy, refined sweets, processed foods, and artificial chemicals. These foods are known to upset the body's natural balance and may worsen chronic health disorders. Individuals who exclude or limit acidic items from their diet can reduce inflammation, boost detoxification, and produce a more alkaline internal environment conducive to healing.

### 3. Use Herbal Remedies:

Dr. Sebi recommended herbal treatments to supplement his alkaline diet and promote healing. Herbs like burdock root, dandelion, sarsaparilla, and bladderwrack are thought to have detoxifying, anti-inflammatory, and immunity-boosting properties. These herbs can be consumed/taken in different ways, including teas, tinctures, capsules, and as part of meals, to boost their medicinal advantages and promote general health and well-being.

### 4. Regular Hydration and Hygiene:

Dr. Sebi underlined the need for regular hydration and hygiene to sustain maximum health. Drinking plenty of clean, alkaline water helps eliminate toxins from the body and supports cellular activity. Additionally, adopting excellent hygiene, such as regular bathing and skin care, aids in the removal of pollutants from the skin and promotes general detoxification.

In essence, a Dr. Sebi-approved diet focuses on alkaline-rich, plant-based meals while avoiding acidic things, combining herbal therapies, and maintaining good hydration and hygiene measures. Individuals who follow these dietary rules and lifestyle recommendations can help their bodies heal naturally and experience increased vitality and well-being.

# HERBAL REMEDIES AND NATURAL HEALING

## An Overview of Dr. Sebi's Recommended Herbal Remedies

Herbal treatments have long been recognized for their medicinal characteristics and capacity to aid in natural healing processes. Dr. Sebi, a proponent of holistic medicine, frequently prescribed certain herbs and plants as part of his approach to wellness. These herbal treatments are thought to have special healing capabilities that can alleviate a variety of health issues and boost general well-being.

## 1. Burdock Root (Arctium lappa):

This cleansing herb has been used in traditional medicine for generations. It is high in antioxidants, vitamins, and minerals, making it an excellent supplement to any natural healing plan. Burdock root is thought to improve liver function, enhance digestion, and purify the blood, making it a good detox and cleansing agent.

## 2. Dandelion (Taraxacum officinale):

This cleansing herb has been used medicinally for ages. It contains high content of vitamins C, A, & K, as well as minerals, including potassium, iron, calcium, & potassium. Dandelion is well known for its diuretic effects, which aid in the removal of toxins from the body while also supporting kidney and liver function. Dandelion may also assist digestion, reduce inflammation, and improve immunological function.

## 3. Sarsaparilla (Smilax spp.):

Sarsaparilla (Smilax spp.) is a tropical plant known for its anti-inflammatory and antioxidant benefits. It has historically been used to cure a variety of maladies, including skin conditions, arthritis, and respiratory problems. Sarsaparilla is thought to aid in detoxification, boost immunological function, and increase overall vigor. It may also contain adaptogenic characteristics, which help the body deal with stress and restore balance.

## 4. Bladderwrack (Fucus vesiculosus):

This herb is a seaweed noted for its high iodine content and potential health benefits. It is frequently used to improve thyroid function, control metabolism, and aid in weight loss. Bladderwrack is also thought to have anti-inflammatory, antioxidant, and immune-boosting qualities, making it an important ingredient in herbal therapies for overall health.

Dr. Sebi's natural healing technique included a range of herbal therapies. These herbs are appreciated for their cleansing, anti-inflammatory, antioxidant, and immune-boosting characteristics and can be used as part of a holistic wellness regimen to promote overall health and vitality.

## Healing Properties of Specific Herbs and Plants

Herbs and plants have long been valued for their medicinal characteristics and powerful healing benefits on the body. Dr. Sebi's approach to natural treatment frequently includes the use of certain herbs and plants, each appreciated for its distinct therapeutic characteristics and potential to promote total well-being.

**1. Burdock Root (Arctium lappa):** This herb is known for its cleansing capabilities and potential to improve liver function. Burdock root is high in antioxidants, which help eliminate toxins from the blood & lymphatic systems, supporting bright skin and overall health. Burdock root also includes anti-inflammatory chemicals that may relieve arthritis symptoms and improve digestive health by promoting bile production.

**2. Dandelion (Taraxacum officinale):** This herb is known for its diuretic and liver-supportive benefits. It promotes detoxification by boosting urine production, removing toxins from the kidneys, and improving liver function. Dandelion is also high in vitamins A, C, & K, and also minerals like calcium, & iron, making it a nutritious addition to any herbal regimen. Its anti-inflammatory effects may also aid to ease arthritic symptoms and improve intestinal health.

3. **Sarsaparilla (Smilax spp.)**: This herb is known for its anti-inflammatory, antioxidant, and immune-boosting benefits. It has long been used to treat skin disorders, joint pain, and breathing problems. Sarsaparilla may aid in detoxification by improving liver function and encouraging the removal of toxins from the body. Furthermore, its adaptogenic characteristics assist the body in dealing with stress and restoring equilibrium, boosting overall vigor and wellbeing.

**4. Bladderwrack (Fucus vesiculosus):** This herb is a seaweed high in iodine that promotes thyroid health and metabolism. It also contains antioxidants, vitamins, and minerals that improve general health. Bladderwrack's anti-inflammatory characteristics may assist to reduce inflammation in the body, while its immuno-boosting benefits promote a healthy immune system. Additionally, bladderwrack's high fiber content helps digestive health and cleansing by encouraging regular bowel movements.

In summary, specific herbs and plants such as burdock root, dandelion, sarsaparilla, and bladderwrack provide a wide range of medicinal characteristics that aid in detoxification, enhance liver and digestive health, reduce inflammation, and increase overall vitality. Incorporating these herbs into a holistic wellness regimen can help boost the body's natural healing processes and promote long-term health and well-being.

# PART TWO: TREATING SPECIFIC CHRONIC DISEASES

## HEALING DIABETES WITH DR. SEBI'S METHODS

### Understanding the Root Causes of Diabetes

Diabetes is a complex metabolic illness defined by elevated blood sugar levels caused by insufficient insulin synthesis (Type 1) or the body's poor use of insulin (Type 2). Dr. Sebi's holistic approach to diabetes treatment entails identifying & resolving the underlying causes of the problem.

## 1. Insulin Resistance and Beta Cell Dysfunction:

Type 2 diabetes is as a result of insulin resistance and beta cell dysfunction. The pancreas produces/makes insulin, a hormone that helps regulate blood sugar levels by enabling glucose uptake into cells. However, in those with insulin resistance, the cells become less receptive to insulin's effects, resulting in high blood sugar levels.

Over time, the pancreas may fail to generate enough insulin to overcome this resistance, resulting in elevated blood sugar levels and diabetes. Additionally, in Type 1 diabetes, the immune system mistakenly assaults & destroys insulin-producing beta cells in the pancreas, resulting in insulin shortage and hyperglycemia.

## 2. Genetic Predisposition:

Genetic factors can increase/elevate a person's risk of acquiring diabetes. Certain genetic variations may predispose people to insulin resistance, beta cell malfunction, or autoimmune death of beta cells. While genetics alone do not predict diabetes, they can combine with environmental factors like nutrition, physical activity, and obesity to enhance vulnerability to the illness.

## 3. Lifestyle Factors:

Diet, physical activity, & obesity all contribute to the development and progression of diabetes. A diet that is high in refined carbs, processed foods, & bad fats can lead to insulin resistance, obesity, and metabolic dysfunction. Sedentary lifestyles and a lack of exercise enhance the risk factors. Furthermore, obesity, particularly excess abdominal fat, is closely linked to insulin resistance & Type 2 diabetes.

Understanding the underlying causes of diabetes is critical to establishing effective prevention and treatment measures. Dr. Sebi's holistic approach addresses these underlying causes through dietary treatments, lifestyle changes, and herbal medicines targeted at restoring body balance and promoting optimal blood sugar control. Diabetes can be effectively managed and problems avoided by addressing insulin resistance, improving pancreatic function, and promoting general health and vitality.

## Dr. Sebi's Dietary Recommendations and Herbal Remedies for Diabetes

Dr. Sebi's holistic approach to diabetes treatment focuses on dietary changes and herbal therapies that try to restore physiological balance and promote optimal blood glucose management. Individuals can improve pancreas function, reduce inflammation, and increase insulin sensitivity by including specific foods and herbs into their diet.

## 1. Alkaline-Rich Diet:

Dr. Sebi recommends an alkaline-rich diet based on natural, plant-based foods to treat diabetes. This contains a variety of fruits, vegetables, nuts, seeds, and whole grains that are both alkaline-forming and nutrition-packed. These foods assist to keep blood sugar constant, increase satiety, and supply critical vitamins, minerals, and antioxidants for overall health.

## 2. Avoid Acidic Foods:

Processed foods, refined sugars, animal products, and fried foods can cause inflammation, insulin resistance, and blood sugar abnormalities. Dr. Sebi recommended avoiding these acidic chemicals and instead focusing on full, unprocessed foods to lower the risk of diabetes problems and improve metabolic health.

### 3. Herbal Remedies:

In addition to dietary adjustments, Dr. Sebi suggested herbal medicines to help manage diabetes. Certain herbs have been demonstrated to reduce blood sugar levels and improve pancreatic health. Bitter melon, fenugreek, cinnamon, and gymnema sylvestre are typical herbs used to control blood sugar levels, enhance insulin sensitivity, & lower the risk of diabetes complications.

### 4. Hydration and Detoxification:

Dr. Sebi emphasizes the importance of proper hydration and cleansing when managing diabetes. Drinking plenty of clean, alkaline water helps to remove toxins from the body, supports renal function, and promotes cellular health. Additionally, occasional fasting and herbal cleanses can help with detoxification, inflammation reduction, and metabolic function, all of which contribute to better blood sugar control.

In summary, Dr. Sebi's dietary suggestions and herbal therapies for diabetes are aimed at improving pancreas function, lowering inflammation, and increasing general health and vitality. Individuals who follow an alkaline-rich diet, avoid acidic foods, use herbal therapies, and prioritize hydration and cleansing can effectively control diabetes and improve their quality of life.

# MANAGING HIGH BLOOD PRESSURE THE DR. SEBI WAY

## Understanding Hypertension and Its Complications

Hypertension, often known as high blood pressure, is a chronic medical disorder marked by excessive blood pressure in the arteries. Dr. Sebi's approach to high blood pressure management focuses on identifying the underlying causes of hypertension and correcting them through dietary changes, lifestyle adjustments, and herbal therapies.

## 1. Blood Pressure Basics:

Blood pressure is simply defined as the force of circulating blood against artery walls. It is often measured in millimeters of mercury (mmHg) and has two components: systolic pressure (pressure when the heart beats) and diastolic pressure (pressure when the heart rests between beats). Normal blood pressure is normally less than 120/80 mmHg. Hypertension is diagnosed when blood pressure continuously surpasses this level.

## 2. Causes of Hypertension:

Genetics, lifestyle, and medical problems can all contribute to hypertension. Obesity, sedentary lifestyle, high salt intake, excessive alcohol consumption, smoking, stress, and a hypertensive family history are all risk factors. Furthermore, some medical disorders, such as kidney disease, diabetes, and sleep apnea, can raise the risk of hypertension.

## 3. Complications of Hypertension:

Untreated or poorly controlled hypertension can cause major health issues such as eye loss, stroke, heart disease, kidney damage, and vascular dementia. High blood pressure can cause damage the arteries over time, resulting in atherosclerosis (artery hardening and constriction), which raises/increases the risk of heart attack & stroke. Hypertension can also stress the heart and kidneys, resulting in organ damage and dysfunction.

## 4. Lifestyle Modifications:

Dr. Sebi emphasizes the need of lifestyle changes for managing high blood pressure. This involves eating a balanced nutritious diet rich in alkaline-forming foods, minimizing salt intake, keeping a healthy weight, engaging in regular physical exercise/activity, managing stress, quitting smoking, and consuming alcohol in moderation. These lifestyle adjustments can help lower blood pressure and lessen the risk of hypertension-related problems.

To summarize, knowing hypertension and its repercussions is critical for successfully controlling high blood pressure. Individuals can improve blood pressure control, lower their risk of problems, and boost overall cardiovascular health by treating the underlying causes of hypertension and applying Dr. Sebi's lifestyle recommendations.

## Dr. Sebi's Dietary and Lifestyle Recommendations for Managing High Blood Pressure

Dr. Sebi's comprehensive approach to high blood pressure management focuses on dietary and lifestyle changes that reduce inflammation, improve cardiovascular health, and promote general well-being. Individuals who incorporate specific diets and activities into their daily lives can effectively manage hypertension and lower the risk of problems.

**1. Alkaline-Rich Diet:**

Dr. Sebi recommends an alkaline-rich diet with natural, plant-based foods to improve cardiovascular health and blood pressure regulation. Fruits, vegetables, nuts, seeds, & whole grains are alkaline-forming foods high in important nutrients, antioxidants, and fiber. These nutrients help to minimize inflammation, improve blood vessel health, and maintain normal blood pressure levels.

**2. Limit Salt Intake:**

Excess sodium can cause fluid retention and increased blood volume, contributing to high blood pressure levels. Dr. Sebi suggests lowering your salt intake by avoiding processed and packaged meals, which are generally rich in sodium. Instead, people can increase the flavor of their meals with herbs, spices, and natural seasonings without jeopardizing their cardiovascular health.

### 3. Stay Hydrated:

Adequate hydration is crucial for maintaining blood volume and supporting cardiovascular health. Dr. Sebi recommends drinking enough of clean, alkaline water throughout the day to stay hydrated and maintain healthy blood pressure levels. Adequate hydration also aids in the removal of toxins from the body and promotes kidney function, all of which contribute to general health and well-being.

### 4. Engage in Regular Exercise:

Regular exercise/activities can help manage high blood pressure by strengthening the heart, improving circulation, and promoting cardiovascular health. Dr. Sebi recommends 30 minutes of moderate-intensity activity every day, such as walking, swimming, cycling, or yoga. Exercise not only lowers blood pressure, but it also relieves stress, promotes weight loss, and improves mood and sleep quality.

## 5. Stress Management:

Chronic stress can cause or lead to high blood pressure and cardiovascular disease. Dr. Sebi recommends people to relieve stress by practicing deep breathing, meditation, yoga, or spending time in nature. These techniques help to reduce cortisol levels, regulate blood pressure, and generate a sense of calm and well-being.

In summary, Dr. Sebi's dietary and lifestyle suggestions for treating high blood pressure include eating an alkaline-rich diet, minimizing salt intake, staying hydrated, exercising regularly, and managing stress efficiently. Individuals who incorporate these behaviors into their daily lives can improve their cardiovascular health, maintain optimal blood pressure levels, & lower the risk of hypertension problems.

# RENAL HEALTH: HEALING KIDNEY DISEASE WITH DR. SEBI'S REMEDIES

## Overview of Kidney Disease and Its Causes

Kidney disease, often known as renal disease, refers to a variety of disorders that decrease kidney function and can result in major health issues. Dr. Sebi's approach to kidney disease treatment focuses on identifying the underlying reasons for renal dysfunction and resolving them through dietary changes, lifestyle adjustments, and herbal therapies.

**1. Kidney Function:**

The kidneys filter waste & surplus fluids from the blood, regulate electrolyte balance, and produce hormones for blood pressure management and red blood cell synthesis. When the kidneys are injured or unable to function effectively, waste products and fluids accumulate in the body, causing different types of health concerns.

**2. Causes of Kidney Disease:**

Various causes can contribute to kidney disease, such as:

**Diabetes:** Uncontrolled diabetes can cause serious harm to the blood vessels in the kidneys, decreasing/lowering their ability to filter waste & maintain fluid balance.

**Hypertension:** High blood pressure can stretch the blood vessels in the kidneys, causing damage over time.

**Chronic Inflammation:** Autoimmune illnesses, infections, and some drugs can cause chronic inflammation in the kidneys, resulting in tissue damage and dysfunction.

**Genetic Factors:** Certain types of kidney disease are genetic and can run in families.

**Obesity:** Excess body weight/fat increases the risk of renal disease by placing strain on the kidneys and causing inflammation.

**Smoking:** Tobacco usage is associated with an increased risk of renal disease and kidney failure.

## 3. Complications of Kidney Disease:

Untreated or poorly managed renal disease can cause major health complications, such as:

**Kidney Failure:** Severe kidney damage can lead to kidney failure, which is a condition in which the kidneys lose their ability to function correctly & require dialysis or kidney transplantation to survive.

Kidney disease increases/encourages the risk of heart disease and stroke because poor kidney function causes high blood pressure, fluid retention, and electrolyte abnormalities.

**Anemia:** A decrease in the production of erythropoietin, a hormone produced by the kidneys, can cause anemia, which is a manifestation of low red blood cell count and exhaustion.

**Bone Disease:** Kidney disease can disturb the body's calcium and phosphorus balance, causing bone loss and an increased risk of fractures.

Kidney/Renal disease is a serious health problem that can have a significant/great impact on overall health & well-being. Understanding the causes and problems of kidney illness allows patients to make proactive efforts to safeguard their renal health and seek suitable treatment and management techniques, such as those indicated by Dr. Sebi.

## Dr. Sebi's Approach to Supporting Kidney Health through Diet and Herbal Remedies

Dr. Sebi's holistic approach to kidney health focuses on dietary changes and herbal therapies that reduce inflammation, promote detoxification, and support normal kidney function. Individuals can nourish their kidneys, relieve stress on these essential organs, and boost overall renal health by integrating specific foods and herbs into their diets.

**1. Alkaline-Rich Diet:**

Dr. Sebi advocates an alkaline-rich diet based on natural, plant-based foods to promote kidney function. Fruits, vegetables, nuts, seeds, & whole grains are examples of alkaline-forming foods that are also high in nutrients. These foods provide vital vitamins, minerals, antioxidants, and phytonutrients that promote kidney function and reduce inflammation. Furthermore, an alkaline diet promotes a good pH equilibrium in the body, which is beneficial to overall health and fitness.

**2. Limit Acidic Foods:**

These foods can increase inflammation and strain on the kidneys, potentially causing kidney damage over time. Dr. Sebi recommends minimizing or eliminating acidic foods including processed meats, refined sugars, animal products, and fried foods. Individuals can enhance renal health by lowering their consumption of certain items.

## 3. Herbal therapies:

In addition to dietary adjustments, Dr. Sebi suggests herbal therapies to support kidney function. Certain herbs have been demonstrated to have diuretic, anti-inflammatory, and detoxifying qualities, which can improve kidney function and overall renal health. Herbs including dandelion root, nettle leaf, parsley, and corn silk are often used to drain toxins from the kidneys, reduce inflammation, and improve bladder function.

## 4. Hydration and Detoxification:

Optimal kidney health and function depend on proper hydration. Dr. Sebi recommends drinking plenty of clean, alkaline water throughout the day to help drain toxins out of the kidneys and stay hydrated. Additionally, fasting and herbal cleanses can help with detoxification, reducing the stress on the kidneys and increasing overall renal health.

In summary, Dr. Sebi's diet and herbal therapies for kidney health are designed to reduce inflammation, promote detoxification, and support normal kidney function. Individuals can support their kidneys and enhance overall renal wellbeing by including alkaline-rich meals, reducing acidic substances, using herbal therapies, and focusing on hydration and detoxification.

# DR. SEBI CURE FOR HERPES

## Understanding Herpes and its Management

Herpes is a common viral infection that is often caused by the herpes simplex virus (HSV), which can produce cold sores in the mouth or genitals. Dr. Sebi's approach to herpes management focuses on understanding the virus's biology, correcting underlying imbalances in the body, & boosting/increasing the immune system's ability to keep the infection at bay.

## 1. Herpes Virus Types:

There are 2 types of herpes viruses: herpes simplex virus type 1 (HSV-1) and HSV-2. HSV-1 usually causes oral herpes, which appears as cold sores or maybe fever blisters around the mouth. HSV-2 primarily causes genital herpes, which is defined by sores or lesions in the genital area. Both varieties of herpes are very contagious and can be spread by coming in close physical contact with an infected person, such as kissing, sexual activity, or sharing personal objects like utensils or towels.

## 2. Symptoms and Transmission:

Herpes infections cause painful blisters or sores followed by stinging, tingling, or burning sensations. Individuals infected with herpes may experience flu-like symptoms such as fever, headache, & enlarged lymph nodes during the first outbreak. Herpes is most contagious during the period of active outbreaks when blisters or sores are prominent, but the virus can also be transferred in the absence of visible symptoms through a process known as asymptomatic shedding.

## 3. Management and Treatment:

While there is no cure for herpes, Dr. Sebi's approach focuses on symptom management, minimizing breakout frequency and severity, and strengthening immune function. This includes dietary adjustments, lifestyle changes, and herbal therapies designed to boost the body's natural defenses against the infection. Dr. Sebi suggests eating an alkaline-rich diet centered mostly on natural, plant-based foods to boost immune function and minimize inflammation. Furthermore, several herbs, such as burdock root, elderberry, and echinacea, are thought to have antiviral qualities that can help fight herpes infections and improve recovery.

## 4. Prevention and Support:

To prevent the spread of herpes, practice safe sex, use condoms when having sex or dental dams during sexual activity, and avoid intimate contact with people during active outbreaks. Supporting immunological health through enough rest, stress management, regular exercise, and right nutrition can all help to lessen the frequency & severity of herpes outbreaks. Furthermore, obtaining emotional assistance from friends, family, or support groups can help people manage with the emotional issues that come with living with herpes.

In summary, herpes is a common viral infection that is mostly caused by the herpes simplex virus that results in painful blisters or sores. While there is no cure for herpes, Dr. Sebi's approach focuses on symptom management, immune function support, and minimizing the frequency and severity of outbreaks through dietary, lifestyle, and herbal therapies.

## Dr. Sebi's Natural Approach to Managing Herpes Outbreaks

Dr. Sebi's comprehensive approach to herpes outbreak management focuses on promoting the body's natural healing mechanisms, fortifying the immune system, and minimizing inflammation. Individuals can alleviate symptoms, minimize the frequency of breakouts, and promote general well-being by making certain food adjustments and lifestyle changes and using herbal therapies.

## 1. Alkaline-Rich Diet:

Dr. Sebi recommends an alkaline-rich diet with plant-based foods to boost immune function and minimize inflammation during herpes outbreaks. Fruits, vegetables, nuts, seeds, & whole grains are high in important nutrients, antioxidants, and phytonutrients and have an alkaline pH. These meals contribute to a good pH balance in the body, aid in detoxification, and promote general health and wellness.

## 2. Herbs and Supplements:

Herbs and supplements with antiviral characteristics may help treat herpes infections and symptoms. Dr. Sebi suggests including herbs like burdock root, elderberry, echinacea, and goldenseal into your diet or taking herbal supplements to boost immune function and lessen the severity of breakouts. Furthermore, supplements containing lysine, an important amino acid, may assist in limiting herpes virus replication and enhance healing.

## 3. Hydration and Detoxification:

Proper hydration supports immunological function, promotes detoxification, and reduces inflammation from herpes outbreaks. Dr. Sebi recommends drinking enough pure, alkaline water all through the day to stay hydrated and promote overall health and wellness. Periodic fasting and herbal cleanses can also help with detoxification, lessen the immune system's burden, and promote internal healing.

## 4. Stress Management:

Stress can weaken the immune system and disturb hormonal balance, leading to herpes outbreaks. Dr. Sebi highlights the need for stress management strategies, including deep breathing, meditation, yoga, and spending time in nature for stress reduction and relaxation. Additionally, regular physical activity, appropriate rest, and mindfulness practice can help decrease stress and promote general well-being.

## 5. Personal Hygiene:

Maintaining good personal cleanliness prevents the transmission of herpes and lowers the chance of recurring outbreaks. Dr. Sebi encourages people to wash their hands frequently, not touch or itch active lesions, and keep the affected region clean and dry. Additionally, using soft, natural soaps and avoiding harsh chemicals or irritants might aid in soothing and protecting the skin during outbreaks.

In summary, Dr. Sebi's advice for naturally controlling herpes breakouts emphasizes immunological function, inflammation reduction, and overall well-being through dietary changes, herbal medicines, hydration, stress management, and basic personal cleanliness. Individuals who incorporate these holistic ways into their daily lives can ease symptoms, lessen the frequency of breakouts, and improve their overall quality of life.

# DR. SEBI CURE FOR HEART DISEASE

## Addressing Heart Disease Risk Factors and Prevention Strategies

Heart disease, often known as cardiovascular disease, refers to different types of disorders that affect the heart and blood arteries, such as coronary artery disease, heart failure, and stroke. Dr. Sebi's approach to treating heart disease is centered on recognizing and managing the underlying risk factors that contribute to the development & progression of cardiovascular disease, as well as implementing preventative techniques to maintain heart health.

### 1. Heart Disease Risk Factors:

Several factors contribute to the development of heart disease, such as:

**Poor Diet:** A diet that contains high refined sugar, processed foods, unhealthy fats, and salt can raise the risk of heart disease by encouraging inflammation, obesity, high blood pressure, and high cholesterol.

**Lack of Physical Activity:** Sedentary lifestyles and a lack of regular exercise increase the risk of obesity, high blood pressure, and poor cardiovascular fitness, all of which lead to heart disease.

**Smoking:** Tobacco smoking is a major contributing risk factor for heart disease because it destroys blood vessels, causes inflammation, and raises the chance of blood clots and plaque development in arteries.

High blood pressure, also known as hypertension, puts strain on the heart and blood arteries, raising the risk of a stroke or heart attack, or heart failure.

High cholesterol: Elevated levels of LDL cholesterol (the "bad" cholesterol) and triglycerides can cause plaque accumulation in the arteries, constricting the blood vessels and raising the risk of heart disease.

Obesity: Excess body weight, particularly visceral fat in the abdomen, raises/increases the risk of heart disease by increasing inflammation, insulin resistance, high blood pressure, and abnormal lipid levels.


2. Prevention Strategies:

Dr. Sebi recommends a comprehensive strategy to preventing heart disease, including:

**Adopting an Alkaline-Rich Diet:** Dr. Sebi suggests an alkaline-rich diet based mostly on natural, plant-based foods to promote heart health and minimize inflammation. This includes fruits, vegetables, nuts, seeds, whole grains, and healthy fats, all of which provide critical nutrients, antioxidants, and fiber that help with cardiovascular function.

**Regular Physical Activity:** Regular physical exercise/activity, such as walking, running, swimming, or cycling, helps to enhance cardiovascular fitness, lower blood pressure, cholesterol levels, and support overall heart health.

**Maintaining a Healthy Weight:** A balanced nutritious diet & regular activity/exercise help to minimize the risk of heart disease by improving insulin sensitivity, reducing inflammation, and enhancing general well-being.

**Quitting Smoking:** Tobacco smoking is a significant modifiable risk factor for cardiovascular disease. Dr. Sebi encourages people to quit smoking and avoid secondhand smoke in order to lower their risk of cardiovascular disease.

**Managing Stress:** Continous stress can contribute to the development and progression of heart disease by raising blood pressure, causing inflammation, and altering the heart rhythm. Dr. Sebi suggests stress-reduction strategies like deep breathing, meditation, yoga, or spending time in nature to increase calm and lower the risk of heart disease.

**3. Herbal Remedies and Supplements:**

Some herbs and supplements are thought to improve heart health & lower/reduce the risk of cardiovascular disease. Dr. Sebi suggests introducing herbs like hawthorn berry, garlic, ginger, and turmeric into your diet or using herbal supplements to boost cardiovascular function, increase blood flow, and reduce inflammation. Supplements like coenzyme Q10, omega-3 fatty acids, and magnesium may also help with heart health and lower the risk of heart disease.

In conclusion, treating heart disease risk factors and implementing preventive methods is critical for improving heart health & lowering the risk of cardiovascular disease. Individuals can support heart health and lower their risk of heart disease by taking a holistic approach that includes dietary changes, regular exercise/activities, stress management, and herbal medicines, which is consistent with Dr. Sebi's natural healing ideas.

# Dr. Sebi's Dietary and Lifestyle Recommendations to Maintain Heart Health

Dr. Sebi's holistic approach to heart health emphasizes on eating a plant-based diet high in alkaline-forming foods, engaging in regular physical activity/exercise, effectively managing stress, & avoiding hazardous substances like tobacco and excessive alcohol. Individuals who address these critical components of their lifestyle can improve cardiovascular function, lower their risk of heart disease, and increase general well-being.

## 1. Alkaline-Rich Diet:

Dr. Sebi recommends an alkaline-rich diet with plant-based foods to promote heart health. Fruits, vegetables, nuts, seeds, whole grains, and healthy fats are all good sources of critical nutrients, antioxidants, and fiber that help with cardiovascular function and inflammation reduction. These foods contribute to a good pH balance in the body, stimulate detoxification, and promote general health and wellness.

## 2. Limit Acidic meals:

Processed meals, refined carbohydrates, unhealthy fats, and high salt intake can cause inflammation and strain on the heart and blood vessels. Dr. Sebi recommends minimizing or eliminating acidic substances and focusing on whole, unprocessed foods to lower the risk of heart disease & also improve cardiovascular health.

## 3. Regular Physical Activity:

Regular exercise promotes heart health and lowers the risk of heart disease. Dr. Sebi suggests incorporating aerobic exercise, weight training, and flexibility exercises into your weekly regimen to enhance cardiovascular fitness, lower blood pressure, cholesterol levels, and increase general well-being.

## 4. Stress Management:

Chronic stress can harm heart health by causing high blood pressure, inflammation, and irregular heartbeat. Dr. Sebi urges people to handle stress efficiently by practicing relaxation techniques including deep breathing, meditation, yoga, and spending time outside. Furthermore, engaging in hobbies, socializing with friends and family, and practicing mindfulness can help reduce stress and improve heart health.

## 5. Avoid Harmful Substances:

Tobacco use increases the risk/probability of heart disease by damaging blood vessels, causing inflammation, and increasing the chance of blood clots & plaque formation in arteries. Dr. Sebi urges people to quit smoking and avoid secondhand smoke to lower their risk of cardiovascular disease. Excessive alcohol intake can also cause high blood pressure, heart rhythm problems, and cardiomyopathy, which affects the heart muscle. Dr. Sebi advocates reducing alcohol use and avoiding binge drinking to improve heart health.

In summary, Dr. Sebi's dietary and lifestyle suggestions for preserving heart health include eating an alkaline-rich diet, engaging in regular physical activity/exercise, effectively managing stress, and avoiding hazardous substances such as tobacco and excessive alcohol. Individuals who include these holistic techniques into their daily lives can improve cardiovascular function, lower their risk of heart disease, and increase general well-being.

# LIFESTYLE PRACTICES FOR LONG-TERM HEALTH

## Advice on Adopting Healthy Lifestyle Habits to Support Long-Term Healing and Wellness

In this chapter, we'll look at Dr. Sebi's advise on developing good lifestyle practices to promote long-term healing and wellness. Dr. Sebi emphasizes the value of comprehensive self-care techniques that address physical, mental, and emotional well-being.

**1. Nutrient-Dense Diet:**

Dr. Sebi recommends a nutrient-dense diet with alkaline-forming foods to promote maximum health. This includes different of fresh fruits, vegetables, nuts, seeds, whole grains, and healthy fats. Individuals who prioritize whole, unprocessed foods can give their bodies with the critical vitamins, minerals, antioxidants, and fiber required for cellular function, immunological support, and general vigor.

## 2. Hydration:

Proper hydration is essential for sustaining good health and promoting natural detoxification processes. Dr. Sebi recommends that you drink enough of clean, alkaline water throughout the day to stay hydrated and enhance cellular hydration. Proper hydration aids in detoxification, digestion, temperature regulation, and overall health.

## 3. Regular Exercise:

Regular exercise promotes cardiovascular health, muscle tone, flexibility, and vitality. Dr. Sebi urges people to engage in regular exercise, such as walking, jogging, swimming, cycling, or yoga, to improve their physical fitness and general well-being. Finding pleasurable activities that encourage mobility and incorporating them into daily life can help people stay active and energized.

## 4. Stress Management:

Chronic stress can negatively impact both physical & mental health, leading to inflammation, hormone imbalances, and reduced immune function. Dr. Sebi recommends that people prioritize stress management strategies like deep breathing, meditation, mindfulness, and spending time in nature to promote relaxation and lessen the effects of stress on the body. Hobbies, socializing with loved ones, and practicing appreciation can all help you develop a good outlook and resilience in the face of life's adversities.

## 5. Quality Sleep:

Regular restorative sleep promotes general health and well-being. Dr. Sebi suggests emphasizing healthy sleep by sticking to a consistent sleep schedule, developing a soothing nighttime routine, and creating a pleasant sleeping environment. Quality sleep boosts immunological function, improves mental clarity, regulates mood, and aids in physical recovery and repair.

## 6. Self-Care Practices:

Provide time for self-care to nourish the mind, body, and spirit. Dr. Sebi recommends people to prioritize self-care activities including journaling, gratitude, spending time in nature, doing hobbies, and connecting with loved ones. These exercises assist to relieve stress, improve emotional well-being, and boost overall health and vitality.

In conclusion, developing good lifestyle behaviors is critical for long-term recovery and wellness. Individuals can support their bodies' natural healing processes and nurture a vibrant and robust state of health by eating nutrient-dense meals, staying hydrated, exercising regularly, managing stress efficiently, getting enough sleep, and practicing self-care.

## Tips for Managing Stress, Incorporating Exercise, and Improving Sleep Quality

In this section, we'll look at Dr. Sebi's practical advice and tactics for reducing stress, incorporating exercise into daily life, and enhancing sleep quality to promote long-term health and wellness.

## 1. Stress Management:

Chronic stress can negatively impact both physical & mental health, causing inflammation, hormone imbalances, and reduced immune function. Dr. Sebi proposes some helpful stress management strategies:

Deep Breathing: Deep breathing exercises might help you relax and reduce stress levels. Take slow, deep breathes in via the nose, hold for a few seconds, and then slowly exhale through your mouth.

Meditation: Incorporate meditation into your everyday practice to relax your mind, alleviate worry, and foster inner serenity. Find a quiet place, sit comfortably, and concentrate on your breathing or a calming mantra.

Mindfulness: Mindfulness involves the practice of being fully present in the moment and nonjudgmentally noticing your thoughts, feelings, and sensations. To develop a greater sense of awareness and present, engage in mindfulness-based daily activities such as eating, walking, or showering.

Nature Therapy: Spending time in nature can help relieve stress, improve mood, and increase general well-being. Take leisurely stroll in the park, spend time gardening, or simply relax outside and enjoy the natural beauty around you.

## 2. Exercise:

Regular physical activity promotes cardiovascular health, muscle tone, and overall well-being. Dr. Sebi suggests incorporating exercise into your regular routine using the following guidelines:

Find Activities You Enjoy: Select activities that you enjoy and look forward to, such as walking, dancing, swimming, cycling, or yoga. Finding activities you enjoy makes exercise feel less like a chore and more like a rewarding experience.

Start cautiously: If you're new to exercising or have been inactive for a long, begin cautiously and gradually increase the intensity and duration of your sessions. To avoid injury & burnout, listen to your body and avoid excessive exercise.

Maintain Consistency: Aim for consistency rather than perfection in your training program. Set realistic goals, stick to a regular schedule, and make exercise a must-do element of your daily routine.

Mix it up: Try out new hobbies and programs to keep your exercise routine fresh. To keep your body challenged and engaged, combine cardiovascular exercise with strength training, flexibility exercises, and mind-body practices.

### 3. Improving Sleep Quality:

Adequate sleep is essential/crucial for overall health and well-being, however many individuals experience sleep disorders. Dr. Sebi recommends the following strategies to improve sleep quality:

Establish a Bedtime Routine: Create a peaceful nighttime routine to alert your body that it's time to unwind and prepare for sleep. This could involve things like taking a warm bath, practicing relaxation techniques, or reading a book.

Create a comfortable sleeping environment: Make effore to ensure your bedroom dark, quiet, and comfy so that you can sleep soundly. Invest in a supportive mattress & pillows, block out light that comes with blackout curtains or an eye mask, and keep the room at a comfortable temperature.

Limit Screen Time: Reduce screen time before bedtime, as blue light from electronic devices can interfere with melatonin production and alter sleep patterns. Instead, try relaxing activities that encourage sleep, such as reading or listening to peaceful music.

Practice relaxation techniques: Use relaxation techniques like muscle relaxation, deep breathing, or guided imagery to calm the mind and body and prepare for sleep. Experiment with several relaxation techniques to determine what works best for you.

Stress management, exercise, and enhancing sleep quality are all important lifestyle behaviors for maintaining long-term health and wellness. Dr. Sebi's advice and tactics can help people create more resilience, energy, and overall well-being in their daily lives.

# NAVIGATING CHALLENGES AND CRITICISMS

## Addressing Common Criticisms and Misconceptions about Dr. Sebi's Healing Methods

In this chapter, we will discuss some of the most common concerns and misconceptions about Dr. Sebi's therapeutic procedures. While Dr. Sebi's approach to health and wellness has gained appeal among those looking for natural alternatives to conventional treatment, it has also been met with criticism and doubt from a variety of sources. Here, we'll look at and clarify some of the most common critiques and misconceptions:

## 1. Lack of Scientific Evidence:

Critics argue that Dr. Sebi's treatment procedures lack scientific data to substantiate their efficacy. Critics believe that many of Dr. Sebi's assertions are unsupported by serious scientific study or clinical studies. However, it is critical to understand that the lack of scientific validation does not rule out the possible benefits of natural healing treatments. Many traditional therapeutic treatments have been utilized for generations, with anecdotal evidence supporting their efficacy, yet they have not been fully examined in Western scientific contexts.

## 2. Claims about "cure-all" remedies:

Another prevalent misconception regarding Dr. Sebi's therapeutic procedures is that they provide a "cure-all" solution for all diseases. While Dr. Sebi's approach stresses holistic healing and correcting fundamental imbalances in the body, it is critical to recognize that no single medicine or treatment can cure all diseases. Healing is a multidimensional process that necessitates personalized approaches adapted to each individual's specific needs and circumstances.

## 3. Allegations of Pseudoscience:

Critics characterize Dr. Sebi's therapeutic procedures as pseudoscience, claiming they lack scientific legitimacy and rely on unproven or questionable ideas. However, it is critical to note that many natural healing techniques, such as herbal medicine, food therapy, and lifestyle treatments, have been used for centuries in a variety of countries and traditions. While some components of Dr. Sebi's approach may contradict current medical paradigms, they are founded on notions of holistic health and natural healing that appeal to many people looking for alternatives to mainstream treatment.

## 4. Commercialization and Profit Motives:

Critics argue that Dr. Sebi and his group benefit from natural healing practices, exploiting vulnerable individuals seeking health remedies. While Dr. Sebi's products and services are marketed and sold to consumers, it is vital to acknowledge that offering access to natural healing treatments and education has expenses. Furthermore, many people have claimed pleasant experiences and health gains as a result of Dr. Sebi's approaches, indicating that his approach may have true worth.

## 5. Lack of Regulation and monitoring:

Dr. Sebi's therapeutic procedures face criticism for a lack of regulation and monitoring in their manufacture and dissemination. Critics claim that without strong quality control standards and uniform testing, consumers may be harmed by unregulated or tainted items. While customers must exercise caution and skepticism when purchasing health goods, it is equally critical to understand that not all natural cures require the same level of regulation as pharmaceutical pharmaceuticals.

In conclusion, while Dr. Sebi's therapeutic methods have received criticism and doubt from numerous sources, they have also received support and praise from many people who have seen great results. By addressing frequent complaints and misconceptions with clarity and candor, we can build a more nuanced knowledge of Dr. Sebi's approach to health and wellness, empowering people to make educated decisions about their health.

## Strategies for Overcoming Challenges and Staying Committed to the Healing Journey

Going on a therapeutic path, especially one that deviates from traditional medical techniques, can present a number of problems and barriers. In this section, we'll look at how to overcome these obstacles and stay dedicated to the healing journey, even in the face of criticism or skepticism.

### 1. Education and Empowerment:

Education is a powerful instrument to overcome problems and critiques. Take the time to explore and comprehend the ideas that underpin Dr. Sebi's treatment approaches, such as the significance of diet, lifestyle, and natural remedies in promoting health and wellness. By learning about the potential benefits and limitations of natural healing, you might feel more empowered to make informed decisions about your health.

## 2. Seek Support and Community:

Experiencing doubt or criticism from others can lead to feelings of isolation during the healing process. Seek out helpful communities and like-minded people who share your views and principles about natural health. Connecting with others who understand & validate your experiences, whether through online forums, support groups, or local gatherings, may be invaluable in terms of support and encouragement.

### 3. Maintain an Open-Minded and adaptable Approach:

Being devoted to your healing path is crucial, but so is remaining open-minded and adaptable. Healing is a dynamic and individualized process, so what works for one person may not work for another. Be open to experimenting, adapting, and adjusting your approach to meet your specific requirements and experiences.

## 4. Practice Self-Compassion:

Healing involves patience, tenacity, and compassion. Be kind with yourself and recognize that growth may be gradual and nonlinear. Celebrate tiny accomplishments, exercise self-care, and develop self-compassion for oneself, especially during difficult circumstances. Remember that healing is a lifetime journey, not a destination, and it is acceptable to take breaks, rest, and recharge as needed.

## 5. Focus on Personal Growth and Empowerment:

See your recovery path as an opportunity for personal growth, empowerment, and self-discovery. Accept obstacles as chances for learning and progress, and build resilience in the face of adversity. You may overcome obstacles with confidence and resilience if you prioritize personal empowerment and take charge of your health and wellness.

## 6. Trust Your Intuition:

Try relying on your inner wisdom to guide you through your recovery path. Listen to your body, respect your instincts, and believe that you know what's best for you. Tune into your inner guidance system and let it direct you in making decisions that are consistent with your values, beliefs, and aspirations for healing and wellness.

To summarize, overcoming problems and criticism on the healing road necessitates a combination of education, support, openness, self-compassion, empowerment, and trust in one's intuition. Individuals who cultivate these skills and tactics can remain devoted to their path of healing and empowerment despite hurdles and doubt from others.

# EMPOWERING READERS TO TAKE CONTROL OF THEIR HEALTH

## Encouragement for Readers to Take Proactive Steps towards Their Health and Well-being

In this last chapter, we hope to inspire and motivate readers to take active measures toward recovering their health and well-being. Throughout this book, we've looked at the fundamentals of Dr. Sebi's therapeutic methods, the difficulties of navigating criticism, and solutions for staying dedicated to the recovery process. Now it's time to put those ideals into practice and take responsibility of our health.

## 1. You Have the Power:

Recognize your ability to influence your health results. While external conditions and situations can have an impact on your health, the decisions you make on a daily basis have a huge role in deciding your overall well-being. By taking responsibility for your health and adopting a proactive mindset, you may empower yourself to make positive changes and control your health destiny.

## 2. Begin Where You Are:

Improving your health does not necessitate drastic lifestyle changes. Instead, focus on making modest, doable moves in the correct direction. Begin where you are, with the resources and expertise you already have, and progressively expand your efforts over time. Remember that growth is a lifelong journey, not a destination, and every step you take toward greater health is important.

### 3. Prioritize Self-Care:

Self-care is essential for preserving health and well-being. Prioritize self-care activities that feed and nurture your mind, body, and spirit. This may include regular activities/exercise, a healthy diet, appropriate sleep, effective stress management, and mindfulness and relaxation practices. Making self-care a priority in your everyday life allows you to restore your energy reserves and cope better with the pressures of modern existence.

### 4. Educate Yourself:

Knowledge is power in health and wellness. Take the time to learn about nutrition, natural healing methods, and holistic approaches to wellness. Stay up to date on the newest research and innovations in integrative medicine, and be willing to consider various points of view. By arming yourself with knowledge, you can make more educated health decisions and advocate for your own well-being.

## 5. Seek Support and responsibility:

Recognize the importance of seeking support and responsibility during your health journey. Whether it's joining a support group, working with a health coach, or enlisting the help of friends and family, being surrounded by a supportive community can provide encouragement, motivation, and advice along the journey. Having someone to share your problems and accomplishments with might make the path to better health seem less onerous and more doable.

## 6. Trust Your Intuition:

Listen to your body, respect your instincts, and believe that you know what's best for you. Tune in to your inner guidance system and let it direct you in making decisions that are consistent with your values, beliefs, and health and well-being goals. By placing your trust in yourself and your inner intelligence, you can boldly take control of your health and live a vigorous and fulfilling life.

Encouraging readers to take responsibility of their health necessitates adopting a proactive mindset, prioritizing self-care, educating oneself, seeking help, and following one's instinct. By adopting these ideas into their daily lives, readers can embark on a journey to optimal health and well-being, empowering them to live the vibrant, meaningful lives they desire.

## CONCLUSION

In conclusion, "Dr. Sebi Cure for All Diseases" provides a thorough guide to implementing Dr. Sebi's holistic approach to health and well-being. Throughout this book, we've looked at Dr. Sebi's therapeutic philosophy, concepts, and natural approaches to treating chronic conditions. This book provides readers with practical ideas and tactics for recovering their health, including understanding the core causes of illnesses, applying dietary modifications, using herbal medicines, and navigating hurdles along the recovery process.

This book hopes to motivate people to embark on their own healing journeys with confidence and determination by encouraging them to take control of their health and giving opportunities for more learning and assistance. Whether you are suffering from diabetes, cancer, high blood pressure, kidney disease, herpes, heart disease, or any other chronic illness, Dr. Sebi's healing methods provide a holistic and natural approach to wellness that centers on addressing the root causes of disease and promoting overall vitality.

Remember that healing is a process that involves patience, perseverance, and self-compassion. Trust your body's intrinsic healing power and take proactive actions to nourish your mind, body, and spirit. Surround yourself with supportive communities, seek advice from qualified practitioners, and remain open to new opportunities for healing and growth.

Finally, I'd like to convey my heartfelt gratitude to all of the readers who have joined me on this journey. Thank you for being open, curious, and dedicated to regaining your health and well-being. May this book be a guiding light on your path to good health, vitality, and well-being. Remember that you have the ability to alter your health and lead a life of prosperity and energy. Here's to a healthy, happy, and healing path ahead.

Made in the USA
Columbia, SC
22 October 2024